# LEAN AND HEALTHY CODES

*A Comprehensive Meal Plan for Rapid Weight Loss and Beating Obesity, Infused with Exercise Strategies for Maximum Results.*

**By Kayren K. Mariirk**

# TABLE OF CONTENT

# INTRODUCTION

Picture this: You, stepping onto the scale, witnessing the numbers drop with each passing day. Your clothes fitting better, your energy soaring, and your confidence radiating from within. It's not just a dream – it's your reality with our groundbreaking weight loss program.

Meet Mark, who once felt trapped in a body he didn't recognize. But with determination and the guidance found in this book, he reclaimed his health and lost an astounding 30kg in just two months. His journey is a testament to the transformative power of belief and action.

Ready to embark on your own journey of transformation? Don't let another day go by without taking the first step towards the life you deserve. Join Mark and countless others who have discovered the power within "lean and healthy." Your future self is waiting – seize it now!

Dear Reader,

Welcome on the path to a happier, healthier version of yourself! Whether you've just decided to embark on this transformative path or you're already well on your way, I want to extend a heartfelt welcome and commend you for taking this courageous step towards reclaiming your health.

In the pages of this book, you'll find a roadmap designed specifically to help you shed a reasonable amount of weight in just a short time. It's not just about losing weight; it's about gaining confidence, vitality, and a renewed zest for life.
Throughout this journey, remember that you're not alone. I promise to be by your side at every turn, offering you advice, encouragement, and support. Together, we'll navigate the ups and downs, celebrate your victories, and overcome any obstacles that may arise.

So, let's embark on this journey together with determination, resilience, and an unwavering commitment to your well-being. Get ready to discover delicious recipes, practical meal plans, effective exercise strategies, and invaluable tips for sustainable success.

Believe in yourself, trust the process, and remember that every small step forward is a triumph. You have the power to transform your life, and I'm honored to be a part of your journey.

With warmest regards,

Kayren K. Mariirk

# ABOUT THE AUTHOR

Concerning the Writer Kayren K. Mariirk is a passionate wellness enthusiast with a background in holistic health practices and a lifelong dedication to personal wellness. She is committed to assisting people in reaching their weight reduction objectives and also living healthy. Mariirk, who has years of experience in the fitness and health sector, blends knowledge with compassion to provide practical weight-loss plans that last. She is also deeply committed to empowering others, a firm believer in the transformational potential of a healthy diet and way of living. Mariirk hopes to encourage and assist readers in their pursuit of a happier, healthier life through this book.

# CHAPTER 1: UNDERSTAND WEIGHT LOSS

Weight loss is a journey that many embark on with various goals in mind, whether it's to improve health, boost confidence, or enhance overall well-being. However, achieving weight loss requires more than just a desire to shed pounds—it requires an understanding of the fundamental principles that govern the process.

## THE BASICS OF WEIGHT LOSS

Let's delve into the basics of weight loss to gain insight into how our bodies respond to different factors and how we can effectively manage our weight.

**Caloric Balance**: At its core, weight loss is about creating a caloric deficit, which means consuming fewer calories than your body expends. This deficit forces the body to tap into its fat stores for energy, resulting in weight loss over time.

Understanding the concept of caloric balance is essential for anyone looking to shed excess weight.

**Nutrition**: The foods we eat play a crucial role in determining our weight and overall health. A balanced diet that includes a variety of nutrient-rich foods, such as fruits, vegetables, lean proteins, whole grains, and healthy fats, is essential for supporting weight loss efforts. By focusing on nutrient-dense foods, we can nourish our bodies while also managing our calorie intake.

**Exercise**: Physical activity is another key component of weight loss. Regular exercise not only burns calories but also helps build lean muscle mass, which can increase metabolism and improve overall body composition. Finding enjoyable forms of exercise, whether it's walking, running, cycling, or dancing, can make it easier to stay active and consistent with your workouts.

**Metabolism**: The body's process of turning food into energy is known as metabolism. A faster metabolism can help burn calories more efficiently, making weight loss easier to achieve. While factors such as genetics and age influence metabolism, certain strategies, such as strength training and consuming protein-rich foods, can help boost metabolism and support weight loss efforts.

**Hydration**: Staying hydrated is crucial for overall health and can also support weight loss. Drinking an adequate amount of water helps maintain proper bodily functions, promotes satiety, and can even boost metabolism. To help you keep hydrated and achieve your weight loss objectives, make it a point to drink a lot of water throughout the day.

**Sleep**: Sleep: Quality sleep is frequently disregarded, although it plays an important role in weight loss and overall health. A lack of sleep can affect hormonal balance, increase appetite, and impede weight loss efforts. Prioritize getting enough sleep each night to support your body's natural processes and optimize weight loss.

**Mindset**: Lastly, adopting a positive mindset is essential for long-term weight loss success. Maintaining a positive outlook, setting realistic goals, and practicing self-compassion can help you stay motivated and resilient in the face of challenges. Remember that weight loss is an ongoing process, and improvement is not necessarily linear. Celebrate your successes, learn from setbacks, and keep moving forward with determination and perseverance.

In conclusion, weight loss is a multifaceted process that involves managing calorie intake, prioritizing nutrient-rich foods, staying active supporting

**Be Specific:** Instead of setting vague goals like "lose weight," get specific about what you want to achieve. How much weight do you want to lose? By when? Setting clear and measurable goals helps keep you focused and accountable.

**Break it down:** Large goals can be overwhelming, so divide them into smaller, more attainable milestones Celebrate each milestone along the way—it's all about progress, not perfection!

**Set Realistic Timelines**: Rome wasn't built in a day, and neither is sustainable weight loss. Be realistic about the time it will take to reach your goals. Aim for steady, gradual progress rather than quick fixes or crash diets.

**Consider Your Lifestyle:** Your weight loss goals should align with your lifestyle, preferences, and priorities If you love dessert, don't deprive yourself completely—find ways to enjoy treats in moderation while still making progress towards your goals.

**Be Flexible:** Life happens, and it's okay to adjust your goals as needed. Be flexible and willing to adapt your plan based on your progress, setbacks, and changing circumstances.

**Focus on Non-Scale Victories**: While the number on the scale is one measure of progress, it's not the only one. Celebrate non-scale victories like increased energy, improved mood, and better sleep—they're just as important!

**Stay Positive:** Finally, keep a positive attitude and believe in yourself. Remember that setbacks are a natural part of any journey, and they don't define your worth or ability to succeed. Stay focused, stay motivated, and most importantly, be kind to yourself along the way.In conclusion, setting realistic goals is essential for long-term success in your weight loss journey. By being specific, breaking down your goals, setting realistic timelines, aligning with your lifestyle, staying flexible, celebrating non-scale victories, and maintaining a positive mindset, you can set yourself up for success and achieve your health and wellness goals. You've got this!

# IMPORTANCE OF NUTRITION IN WEIGHT LOSS

Nutrition plays a vital role in any weight loss journey, serving as the foundation for achieving and maintaining a healthy body weight. Here's why it's so important:

**Calorie Control:** Nutrition directly impacts your calorie intake, which is a key factor in weight loss. By choosing nutrient-dense, low-calorie foods, you can create a calorie deficit necessary for shedding pounds. Incorporating plenty of fruits, vegetables, lean proteins, and whole grains into your diet can help you feel full and satisfied while keeping your calorie intake in check.

**Balanced Macronutrients:** Protein, carbohydrates, and fats are the three macronutrients that provide energy and support various bodily functions. A balanced diet that includes all three macronutrients in appropriate proportions is essential for overall health and weight loss. Protein, in particular, is crucial for preserving lean muscle mass during weight loss and promoting feelings of fullness.

**Nutrient Density**: Nutrient-dense foods are rich in essential vitamins, minerals, and antioxidants that support overall health and well-being. Focusing on nutrient-dense foods like fruits, vegetables, whole grains, and lean proteins ensures that you're providing your body with the essential nutrients it needs to function optimally while also supporting your weight loss goals.

**Blood Sugar Regulation**: Eating a balanced diet that includes complex carbohydrates, fiber, and protein helps regulate blood sugar levels and prevents spikes and crashes in energy levels. Stable blood sugar levels can help reduce cravings, prevent overeating, and support weight loss efforts.

**Satiety and Hunger Management:** Certain foods have been shown to promote feelings of fullness and satiety, which can help control hunger and prevent overeating. High-fiber foods, lean proteins, and healthy fats are particularly effective at promoting satiety and keeping hunger at bay, making it easier to stick to your calorie goals and avoid unnecessary snacking.

**Energy Levels and Performance:** Proper nutrition provides the energy your body needs to fuel physical activity and daily tasks. Eating a well-balanced diet that includes a variety of nutrient-rich foods can help optimize energy levels, improve physical performance, and enhance motivation to stay active—all of which are essential for successful weight loss.

**Long-Term Health:** Beyond weight loss, nutrition plays a crucial role in overall health and disease prevention. Adopting healthy eating habits during your weight loss journey can have long-lasting benefits, reducing the risk of chronic diseases such as heart disease, diabetes, and certain cancers.

By prioritizing nutrient-dense foods, balancing macronutrients, regulating blood sugar levels, managing hunger and satiety, optimizing energy levels, and supporting long-term health, you can achieve sustainable weight loss while nourishing your body from the inside out.

# CHAPTER 2: CREATING A SOLID FOUNDATION

Building a strong foundation is essential for success in any weight loss journey. Here's how to lay the groundwork for lasting results:

1. **Set Clear Goals:** Define your weight loss goals, including how much weight you want to lose and by when. Ascertain that your objectives are time-bound, relevant, quantifiable, attainable, and specific (SMART).

2. **Educate Yourself:** Learn about nutrition, exercise, and behavior change to make informed decisions about your health. Understand the basics of calorie balance, macronutrients, portion control, and the importance of regular physical activity.

3. **Create a Plan:** Develop a personalized plan that includes a balanced diet, regular exercise, adequate sleep, stress management, and other healthy habits. Consider seeking guidance from a healthcare professional or certified

nutritionist to create a plan tailored to your needs.

4.  **Build Healthy Habits:** Focus on adopting sustainable lifestyle changes rather than quick-fix solutions. Incorporate nutritious foods, regular exercise, and stress-relieving activities into your daily routine to create lasting habits.

5.  **Track Your Progress:** Keep track of your food intake, physical activity, and progress toward your goals. Use tools like food journals, fitness apps, or wearable devices to monitor your behavior and make adjustments as needed.Stay Consistent: Consistency is key to success. Stick to your plan even when faced with challenges or setbacks. Recall that development takes time and that little steps taken consistently over time yield big rewards.

6.  **Seek Support:** Surround yourself with a supportive network of friends, family, or online communities who can encourage and motivate you along the way. Consider joining a weight loss group or working with a coach to stay accountable and motivated.

7.  **Exercise Self-Compassion:** Treat yourself with kindness as you go. Accept that there will be ups and downs, and When things

don't go as intended, don't be too hard on yourself. Celebrate your successes and learn from your setbacks with a compassionate attitude.

8.  By laying a solid foundation with clear goals, education, planning, healthy habits, consistency, support, and self-compassion, you can set yourself up for success in your weight loss journey.

Remember, it's not just about reaching a number on the scale—it's about cultivating a healthier, happier lifestyle that lasts a lifetime.

# PRINCIPLES OF HEALTHY EATING

Navigating healthy eating habits is essential for sustainable weight loss. Here are key principles to guide you on your journey:

1.  **Focus on Whole Foods:** Emphasize whole, minimally processed foods in your diet. Fruits, vegetables, whole grains, lean meats, and good fats are a few of these. Whole foods are nutrient-dense and provide essential vitamins, minerals, and fiber to support overall health and weight loss.

2.  **Portion Control:** Keep track of how much you consume to avoid overeating. Use

visual cues or measuring tools to help you gauge appropriate portion sizes for different food groups. Half of your plate should be made up of vegetables, 25% should be lean protein, and 25% should be made up of nutritious grains or starchy veggies.

3. **Balance Macronutrients:** Include a balance of carbohydrates, proteins, and fats in each meal to support energy levels, satiety, and overall health. Focus on high-quality sources of each macronutrient, such as complex carbohydrates, lean proteins, and unsaturated fats.

4. **Moderate Sugar and Processed Foods:** Limit your intake of added sugars, refined grains, and processed foods, which can contribute to weight gain and negatively impact health. Choose whole foods over processed options whenever possible, and be mindful of hidden sugars in packaged foods.

5. **Keep Hydrated:** Drink enough of water throughout the day to preserve your overall health and hydration. Water helps regulate appetite, flush out toxins, and maintain proper bodily functions. Aim to drink at least 8-10 cups of water per day, or more if you're physically active or in hot weather.

6. **Eat Mindfully**: Practice mindful eating by paying attention to your hunger and fullness cues, eating slowly, and savoring each bite. Avoid distractions like TV or screens while eating, and tune into your body's signals to prevent overeating and promote satisfaction.

7. **Include Variety:** Incorporate a variety of foods into your diet to ensure you're getting a wide range of nutrients and flavors. Experiment with different fruits, vegetables, grains, proteins, and cooking methods to keep meals interesting and satisfying.

8. **Plan Ahead:** Plan your meals and snacks ahead of time to avoid spontaneous, unhealthy choices. Stock your kitchen with nutritious foods, prepare meals in advance when possible, and pack healthy snacks to take with you on the go.

9. **Pay Attention to Your Body:** Observe your reactions to various foods and modify your diet accordingly. Choose foods that nourish your body, support your energy levels, and leave you feeling satisfied and energized.

By following these principles of healthy eating, you can fuel your body with the nutrients it needs to support weight loss and overall well-being. Remember that healthy eating is not about deprivation or strict rules—it's about nourishing your body with wholesome foods that promote health and happiness.

# UNDERSTANDING MACRONUTRIENTS

Macronutrients, or "macros," are the key nutrients that provide the majority of the energy (calories) our bodies require to function. Understanding macros is key to achieving your weight loss goals. Let's break down the three main macronutrients—carbohydrates, proteins, and fats—and their roles in supporting weight loss:

**Carbohydrates:**

- Role: Carbs are the body's primary source of energy, providing fuel for muscles, organs, and brain function.

- Types: Carbohydrates are classified into two main categories: simple carbs (sugars) and complex carbs (starches and fibers).

- Weight Loss Tip: Choose complex carbohydrates like whole grains, fruits, and vegetables, which provide sustained energy and fiber to keep you feeling full and satisfied.

**Proteins**:

- Role: Proteins are the building blocks of tissues, muscles, and organs, playing a crucial role in repairing and building new cells.
- Sources: Protein-rich foods include lean meats, poultry, fish, eggs, dairy products, legumes, nuts, and seeds.
- Weight Loss Tip: Prioritize protein-rich foods in your diet to support muscle maintenance and increase feelings of fullness, which can help control appetite and reduce overall calorie intake.

**Fats**:

- Role: Fats are essential for hormone production, cell membrane structure, and the absorption of fat-soluble vitamins (A, D, E, and K).
- Types: Fats are classified into saturated fats, unsaturated fats (monounsaturated and polyunsaturated), and trans fats.
- Weight Loss Tip: Focus on healthy fats from sources like avocados, nuts, seeds, olive oil, and fatty fish. These fats supply critical nutrients and enhance satiety., helping to

control cravings and support weight loss efforts.

To lose weight in a way that will last, your diet must have the proper ratio of macronutrients. Aim to include a variety of nutrient-dense foods from each macronutrient group in your meals and snacks. Balancing your macros can help regulate hunger, support energy levels, and optimize metabolism, ultimately leading to successful weight loss and improved overall health. Remember, it's not just about counting calories—it's about nourishing your body with the right nutrients to fuel your weight loss journey.

# PORTION CONTROL

Portion control refers to the practice of eating a specific amount of food to manage calorie intake and maintain a healthy weight. It involves being mindful of how much food you consume at each meal or snack and ensuring that your portions align with your nutritional needs and weight loss goals.

Here's how portion control works:

**Understanding Serving Sizes:** Portion control starts with understanding recommended serving sizes for different types of foods. Serving sizes are standardized measurements that indicate how much of a particular food constitutes one serving. These serving sizes are typically listed on food packaging and can also be found in nutritional guidelines.

**Measuring and Weighing Food:** One way to practice portion control is by measuring or weighing your food to ensure you're eating the appropriate serving size. You can use measuring cups, kitchen scales, or other portion control tools to accurately portion out your food.

**Using Visual Cues:** In situations where measuring tools are not available, you can rely on visual cues to estimate portion sizes. For example, a portion of beef is around the size of a deck of cards, but a serving of pasta is about the size of a tennis ball. Learning to eyeball portion sizes can help you make healthier choices when dining out or eating at social events.

**Balancing Macronutrients:** Portion control also involves balancing your intake of macronutrients—carbohydrates, proteins, and fats. Aim to include a mix of these macronutrients in each meal to promote satiety, stabilize blood sugar levels, and support overall health.

**Listening to Hunger Cues:** Practicing portion control also means tuning in to your body's hunger and fullness cues. Eat gently and pay attention to how your body feels when eating. To avoid overeating, stop eating when you're satisfied, rather than continuing to eat until you're overly full.

**Preventing Mindless Eating:** Consuming food without thinking, like eating it directly out of a bag or container, might result in overindulgence. Instead, portion out your food onto a plate or bowl before eating to help you control your portions and prevent overindulgence.

Overall, portion control is a valuable tool for managing calorie intake, promoting mindful eating, and supporting weight loss and weight maintenance goals. By being mindful of portion sizes and listening to your body's signals, you can achieve a healthier relationship with food and maintain a balanced diet.

# IMPORTANCE OF PORTION CONTROL

Portion control is a fundamental aspect of successful weight loss. Here's why portion control is essential for achieving and maintaining a healthy weight:

1. You may better regulate how many calories you consume by keeping an eye on portion sizes. Avoiding consumption of excess calories, which can lead to weight gain over time.

2. It prevents overeating, as our bodies may not accurately register when we've consumed enough food. But by sticking to appropriate portion sizes, you can prevent the tendency to overeat and avoid consuming more calories than your body needs.

3. Teaches Mindful Eating: Portion control encourages mindful eating, which involves paying attention to hunger and fullness cues, as well as savoring each bite of food. By eating mindfully, you can better tune in to your body's signals and avoid mindless eating habits, such as eating out of boredom or emotion.

4. Supports Weight Maintenance: Once you've reached your weight loss goals, portion control remains important for weight maintenance. By continuing to eat appropriate portion sizes, you can prevent weight regain and sustain your progress over the long term.

5. Allows Flexibility: Portion control doesn't mean depriving yourself of your favorite foods—it's about enjoying them in moderation. By practicing portion control, you can still enjoy treats and indulgences

while staying within your calorie goals and maintaining a healthy weight.

6. Promotes Awareness: Monitoring portion sizes increases awareness of how much you're eating and can help you make more informed choices about food. Over time, you'll develop a better understanding of appropriate portion sizes and learn to gauge your hunger and fullness more accurately.

In conclusion, portion control is a critical component of successful weight loss and weight maintenance. By managing portion sizes, you can regulate calorie intake, prevent overeating, practice mindful eating, support weight loss goals, and develop a healthier relationship with food. Remember to focus on quality over quantity, savor each bite, and listen to your body's hunger and fullness cues. With portion control as part of your toolkit, you can achieve sustainable weight loss and enjoy a healthier, happier lifestyle.

# CHAPTER 3: THE MEAL PLAN

Dear esteemed reader, below is an organized and well tailored meal plan that you can follow for two months and above, with the aim of losing at least 30kg in two months. To sustain or keep shredding weight after this months you just have to repeat the plan over and over again.

## WEEK 1

| Day | Breakfast | Lunch | Dinner | Snacks |
| --- | --- | --- | --- | --- |
| 1 | 2 scrambled eggs<br>1 cup spinach<br>1/2 cup cherry tomatoes<br>1 | 4 oz grilled chicken breast<br>2 cups mixed Greensburg<br>1/2 cucumber<br>1/2 | 4 oz baked salmon<br>1 cup roasted asparagus<br>1/2 cup cooked quinoa | 1 medium carrot<br>2 tbsp hummus<br>1/2 cup Greek yogurt<br>1 tbsp almonds |

| | | | | |
|---|---|---|---|---|
| | slice whole grain toast | bell pepper<br>2 tbsp balsamic vinaigrette | | |
| 2 | 1 cup oats<br>1/2 sliced banana<br>1 tbsp walnuts | 1 cup lentil soup<br>2 cups mixed greens<br>2 tbsp vinaigrette | 4 turkey meatballs<br>1 cup zucchini noodles<br>1/2 cup marinara sauce | 1 medium apple<br>2 tbsp peanut butter<br>1/2 cup cottage cheese<br>1/2 cup pineapple chunks |
| 3 | 1 cup spinach<br>1/2 | 4 oz grilled chicken | 6 grilled shrimp<br>1/2 | 1/4 cup mixed nuts<br> |

| | | | | |
|---|---|---|---|---|
| | banana<br>1/2 cup almond milk<br>1 scoop protein powder | breast<br>2 cups romaine lettuce<br>2 tbsp Caesar dressing | cup cooked brown rice<br>1 cup steamed broccoli | 1 cup whole grain cereal<br>1/2 cup skim milk |
| 4 | 1/2 cup Greek yogurt<br>1/4 cup mixed berries<br>1 tbsp chia seeds | 4 oz turkey breast<br>1/4 avocado<br>1 whole grain tortilla<br>1 cup mixed vegetables | 4 oz tofu<br>1 cup mixed vegetables<br>1/2 cup cooked brown rice | 1 medium cucumber<br>2 tbsp hummus<br>2 rice cakes<br>1 tbsp almond butter |
| 5 | 1 slice whole | 1 cup black | 4 oz baked | 1/2 cup edamam |

| | | | |
|---|---|---|---|
| grain toast<br>1/4 mashed avocado<br>1 poached egg | beans<br>1/2 cup corn kernels<br>1/4 avocado<br>2 cups mixed greens | cod<br>1 cup roasted Brussels sprouts<br>1/2 cup cooked quinoa | e<br>1 cup spinach<br>1/2 cup pineappl e<br>1/2 cup coconut water |
| 6 | 1/2 cup Greek yogurt<br>1/4 cup granola<br>1/4 cup mixed berries | 4 oz chicken breast<br>1/4 cup spinach<br>1 tbsp feta cheese<br>1/2 cup cooked quinoa | 4 oz tofu<br>1 cup broccoli<br>1/2 cup snap peas<br>1/2 cup cooked brown rice | 1/2 cup Greek yogurt<br>1 tbsp honey<br>1/4 cup trail mix |

| Day | Breakfast | Lunch | Dinner | Snacks |
| --- | --- | --- | --- | --- |
| 7 | 2 whole grain waffles<br>1 tbsp almond butter<br>1/2 cup sliced strawberries | 4 oz chickpeas<br>1/2 cucumber<br>1/2 tomato<br>1/4 cup feta cheese<br>1 tbsp vinaigrette | 6 oz grilled steak<br>1 cup sautéed mushrooms<br>1/2 cup sweet potato mash | 1 scoop protein powder<br>1 cup almond milk<br>1/2 bell pepper<br>1/2 avocado |

## WEEK 2

| Day | Breakfast | Lunch | Dinner | Snacks |
| --- | --- | --- | --- | --- |
| 8 | 2 scrambled eggs<br>1 cup | 4 oz grilled chicken breast<br>1/2 | 4 oz baked tilapia<br>1 cup roasted | 1 medium carrot<br>1/2 cup hummus |

| | | | | |
|---|---|---|---|---|
| | spinach<br>1/2 cup mushrooms | cup mixed vegetables<br>1/2 cup quinoa | vegetables<br>1/2 cup cooked couscous | <br>1/2 cup cottage cheese<br>1/2 cup pineapple chunks |
| 9 | 1 cup oats<br>1/4 cup sliced strawberries<br>1 tbsp chia seeds | 4 oz turkey breast<br>1/4 avocado<br>1 slice whole grain bread | 4 oz grilled chicken breast<br>1 cup steamed broccoli<br>1/2 cup cooked brown rice | 1/2 cup Greek yogurt<br>1/4 cup granola<br>1/2 medium apple<br>1 tbsp almond butter |
| 10 | 1 cup kale<br>1/2 | 1 cup mixed beans<br> | 4 oz baked salmon< | 1/4 cup mixed nuts<br> |

| | | | |
|---|---|---|---|
| | banana<br>1/4 cup mixed berries<br>1 scoop protein powder | r>1/2 cup cherry tomatoes<br>1/2 bell pepper<br>1/4 avocado<br>2 tbsp lime vinaigrette | br>1 cup roasted asparagus<br>1/2 cup cooked quinoa | 1/2 cucumber<br>2 tbsp hummus |
| 11 | 2 slices whole grain toast<br>1/2 mashed avocado<br>2 slices tomato | 1 cup lentil soup<br>2 cups mixed greens<br>2 tbsp vinaigrette | 1 cup turkey chili<br>1 slice whole grain bread | 1/2 cup cottage cheese<br>1/2 cup pineapple chunks<br>2 rice cakes<br |

| | | | | |
|---|---|---|---|---|
| | | | | >2 tbsp hummus |
| 12 | 1/2 cup Greek yogurt<br>1/4 cup granola<br>1/4 cup mixed berries | 4 oz chicken breast<br>1/2 cup mixed vegetables<br>1/2 cup cooked quinoa | 6 grilled shrimp<br>1/2 cup cooked quinoa<br>1 cup sautéed spinach | 1/4 cup mixed nuts<br>1/2 cucumber<br>1/4 cup tzatziki sauce |
| 13 | 1 cup whole grain cereal<br>1/2 cup skim milk<br>1/2 sliced bananas | 2 cups grilled vegetables<br>2 tbsp feta cheese<br>2 tbsp balsamic vinaigrett | 6 oz baked chicken breast<br>1 cup roasted Brussels sprouts<br>1/2 cup | 1/2 cup Greek yogurt<br>1 tbsp honey<br>1/2 medium apple<br>1 tbsp almond |

| Day | Breakfast | Lunch | Dinner | Snacks |
|---|---|---|---|---|
|  |  | e | sweet potato mash | butter |
| 14 | 2 scrambled eggs<br>1 cup spinach<br>1/4 cup feta cheese | 4 oz canned tuna<br>1/2 cup mixed greens<br>1/4 avocado<br>1 whole wheat pita pocket | 4 oz chickpeas<br>1/2 cup mixed vegetables<br>1/2 cup cooked brown rice | 1 medium carrot<br>1/2 cup hummus<br>1/2 cup cottage cheese<br>1/2 cup pineapple chunks |

## WEEK 3

| Day | Breakfast | Lunch | Dinner | Snacks |
|---|---|---|---|---|
| 15 | 1 cup spinach< | 1 cup mixed | 6 oz grilled | 1/4 cup mixed |

| | | | | |
|---|---|---|---|---|
| | br>1/2 banana<br>1/2 cup mango<br>1/2 cup Greek yogurt | beans<br>1/2 cup corn kernels<br>1/4 avocado<br>2 cups mixed greens<br>2 tbsp lime vinaigrette | salmon<br>1 cup cooked quinoa<br>1 cup steamed broccoli | nuts<br>1/2 cucumber<br>1/2 cup hummus |
| 16 | 2 slices whole grain toast<br>1/2 mashed avocado<br>2 slices | 4 oz turkey breast<br>1/2 cup mixed vegetables<br>1/2 cup | 6 oz grilled steak<br>1 cup roasted vegetables<br>1/2 cup cooked | 1/2 cup Greek yogurt<br>1/4 cup mixed berries<br>2 rice cakes<br> |

| | | | | |
|---|---|---|---|---|
| | tomato | cooked brown rice | quinoa | >2 tbsp almond butter |
| 17 | 1 cup oats<br>1/4 cup sliced strawberries<br>1 tbsp almond slices | 4 oz chicken breast<br>2 cups mixed greens<br>1/4 cup croutons<br>2 tbsp Caesar dressing | 6 oz baked chicken thighs<br>1 cup roasted sweet potatoes<br>1 cup green beans | 1/2 cup cottage cheese<br>1/2 cup pineapple chunks<br>2 celery sticks<br>2 tbsp peanut butter |
| 18 | 2 whole grain waffles<br>1 tbsp almond | 4 oz lentils<br>2 cups mixed greens<br>2 | 6 oz grilled salmon<br>1 cup cooked quinoa<b | 1 medium carrot<br>1/2 cup hummus<br>1/2 |

| | | | | |
|---|---|---|---|---|
| | butter<br>>1/2 cup sliced strawberr ies | tbsp vinaigrett e | r>1 cup steamed broccoli | cup cottage cheese< br>1/2 cup |
| 19 | 1/2 cup Greek yogurt<b r>1/4 cup granola< br>1/4 cup mixed berries | 4 oz turkey breast<b r>1/4 avocado <br>2 slices whole grain bread | 6 oz baked chicken breast<b r>1 cup ste | |
| 20 | 1 cup oatmeal< br>1/2 sliced banana< br>1 tbsp chopped | 1 cup lentil soup<br >2 cups mixed greens< br>2 tbsp | 4 oz grilled salmon< br>1 cup roasted asparagu s<br>1/2 cup | 1/4 cup mixed nuts<br> 1 medium carrot<br >1/2 cup hummus |

| | | | |
|---|---|---|---|
| | walnuts | vinaigrette | quinoa | <br>1/2 cup Greek yogurt |
| 21 | 2 scrambled eggs<br>1 cup spinach<br>1/2 cup cherry tomatoes | Turkey and avocado wrap:<br>1 whole wheat tortilla<br>3 oz sliced turkey breast<br>1/4 avocado<br>1/2 cup mixed greens<br>1/4 | 4 oz baked cod<br>1 cup roasted Brussels sprouts<br>1/2 cup cooked brown rice | 1 small orange<br>1/2 cup cottage cheese<br>1/2 cup cucumber slices<br>2 tbsp almond butter |

| | | cup diced tomatoes | | |
| --- | --- | --- | --- | --- |

## WEEK 4

| Day | Breakfast | Lunch | Dinner | Snacks |
| --- | --- | --- | --- | --- |
| 22 | 1 whole grain toast with 1/2 mashed avocado and poached egg | Chickpea salad:<br>1 cup mixed greens<br>1/2 cup chickpeas<br>1/4 cup | 6 oz grilled steak<br>>1 cup sautéed mushrooms and onions<br>1/2 cup sweet | 1/4 cup trail mix<br>1 medium apple<br>>1/2 cup Greek yogurt<br>>1/4 cup grapes |

| | | diced cucumber<br>1/4 cup diced bell pepper<br>2 tbsp feta cheese<br>2 tbsp balsamic vinaigrette | potato mash | |
| 23 | Smoothie: <br>1 cup spinach<br>1/2 banana<br>1/2 cup | Tuna salad: <br>4 oz canned tuna<br>1/4 cup diced celery<br | Veggie stir-fry: <br>4 oz tofu<br>1 cup mixed vegetables<br>1/ | 1/2 cup Greek yogurt with 1/4 cup granola<br>1/2 cup |

| | | | | |
|---|---|---|---|---|
| | mixed berries<br>1/2 cup Greek yogurt | >1/4 cup diced red onion<br>>1 tbsp Greek yogurt<br>1 tsp Dijon mustard<br>1 tbsp lemon juice<br>Salt and pepper to taste | 2 cup cooked quinoa | carrot sticks with hummus |
| 24 | 2 whole grain waffles with 2 tbsp almond butter | Grilled chicken salad:<br>4 oz grilled chicken breast<b | Baked tilapia with roasted vegetables:<br>6 oz | 1/4 cup mixed nuts<br>1 medium apple<br>>1/2 cup |

| | | | | |
|---|---|---|---|---|
| | and sliced strawberries | r>2 cups mixed greens<br>1/4 cup diced cucumber<br>1/4 cup diced bell pepper<br>2 tbsp feta cheese<br>2 tbsp balsamic vinaigrette | tilapia<br>1 cup mixed roasted vegetables (bell peppers, zucchini, onion)<br>1/2 cup quinoa | cottage cheese<br>1/2 cup pineapple chunks |
| 25 | Scrambled eggs with | Lentil soup with | Grilled shrimp skewers | Carrot sticks with |

| | | | | |
|---|---|---|---|---|
| | spinach and mushrooms<br>1 slice whole grain toast | mixed greens salad<br>2 cups mixed greens<br>1/4 cup lentils<br>1/4 cup diced tomato<br>1/4 cup diced cucumber<br>2 tbsp vinaigrette | with brown rice and steamed broccoli<br>6 oz grilled shrimp<br>1/2 cup cooked brown rice<br>1 cup steamed broccoli | hummus<br>1/2 cup Greek yogurt with a sprinkle of almonds |
| 26 | Oatmeal topped with | Turkey and avocado | Veggie and tofu stir-fry | Apple slices with |

| | | | | |
|---|---|---|---|---|
| | sliced bananas and walnuts | sandwich on whole grain bread<br>4 oz sliced turkey breast<br>1/4 avocado<br>2 slices whole grain bread<br>1/2 cup mixed greens | with brown rice<br>4 oz tofu<br>1 cup mixed vegetables<br>1/2 cup cooked brown rice | peanut butter<br>Cottage cheese with pineapple chunks |
| 27 | Smoothie with spinach, banana, almond | Chickpea salad with feta cheese and | Baked cod with roasted Brussels sprouts | Edamame<br>Smoothie made with |

| | milk, and protein powder | balsamic vinaigrette<br>1 cup mixed greens<br>1/2 cup chickpeas<br>2 tbsp crumbled feta cheese<br>2 tbsp balsamic vinaigrette | and quinoa<br>6 oz baked cod<br>1 cup roasted Brussels sprouts<br>1/2 cup cooked quinoa | spinach, pineapple, and coconut water |
| 28 | Greek yogurt with berries | Grilled chicken Caesar salad<br | Grilled steak with sautéed | Mixed nuts<br>Sliced cucumbe |

| and a sprinkle of chia seeds | >4 oz grilled chicken breast<br>2 cups romaine lettuce<br>1/4 cup croutons <br>2 tbsp Caesar dressing | mushrooms and sweet potato mash<br>6 oz grilled steak<br>1 cup sautéed mushrooms<br>1/2 cup sweet potato mash | r with hummus |
| --- | --- | --- | --- |

## WEEK 5



| Day | Breakfast | Lunch | Dinner | Snacks |
| --- | --- | --- | --- | --- |
| 29 | Whole grain toast with mashed avocado and poached eggs | Black bean and corn salad with avocado<br>1/2 cup black beans<br>1/2 cup corn kernels<br>1/4 avocado<br>2 cups mixed greens<br>2 | Baked chicken breast with steamed broccoli and brown rice<br>6 oz baked chicken breast<br>1 cup steamed broccoli<br>1/2 cup cooked brown | Rice cakes with almond butter<br>Apple slices with Greek yogurt |

| | | | | |
|---|---|---|---|---|
| | | tbsp lime vinaigrette | rice | |
| 30 | Chia seed pudding with mixed berries | Quinoa salad with black beans, corn, and avocado<br>1/2 cup cooked quinoa<br>1/4 cup black beans<br>1/4 cup corn kernels<br>1/4 avocado | Baked salmon with asparagus and quinoa<br>6 oz baked salmon<br>1 cup roasted asparagus<br>1/2 cup cooked quinoa | Carrot sticks with hummus<br>Greek yogurt with a drizzle of honey |

| | | | | |
|---|---|---|---|---|
| | | <br>2 cups mixed greens<br>2 tbsp lime vinaigrette | | |
| 31 | Whole grain waffles with almond butter and sliced strawberries | Turkey and vegetable stir-fry with brown rice<br>4 oz sliced turkey breast<br>1 cup mixed vegetables<br>1/ | Grilled shrimp with quinoa and sautéed spinach<br>6 oz grilled shrimp<br>1/2 cup cooked quinoa<br>1 cup | Rice cakes with almond butter<br>Sliced bell peppers with guacamole |

| | | 2 cup cooked brown rice | sautéed spinach | |
|---|---|---|---|---|
| 32 | 2 scrambled eggs<br>1 cup spinach<br>1 slice whole grain toast | Lentil soup: 1 cup<br>Mixed greens salad: 2 cups<br>1/4 cup lentils<br>1/4 cup diced tomato<br>1/4 cup diced cucumber<br>2 tbsp vinaigrett | Grilled chicken breast: 6 oz<br>Mixed roasted vegetables: 1 cup<br>1/2 cup cooked quinoa | Carrot sticks: 1 medium<br>Greek yogurt: 1/2 cup<br>Almonds: 2 tbsp |

| | | e | | |
| --- | --- | --- | --- | --- |
| 33 | 1 cup oats<br>1/2 sliced banana<br>1 tbsp chopped walnuts | Turkey and avocado wrap: 4 oz sliced turkey breast<br>1/4 avocado<br>1 whole grain tortilla<br>1/2 cup mixed greens | Baked cod: 6 oz<br>Quinoa: 1/2 cup<br>Steamed broccoli: 1 cup | Apple slices: 1 medium<br>Peanut butter: 2 tbsp<br>Cottage cheese: 1/2 cup<br>Pineapple chunks: 1/2 cup |
| 34 | Smoothie: 1 cup spinach<br>1/2 banana<br>1/2 | Greek salad with grilled chicken: 4 oz | Stir-fried tofu: 4 oz<br>Mixed vegetables: 1 | Edamame: 1/2 cup<br>Smoothie: 1 cup spinach, |

| | | | |
|---|---|---|---|
| cup almond milk<br>1 scoop protein powder | grilled chicken breast<br>1/2 cup mixed greens<br>1/4 cup diced cucumbe r<br>1/4 cup diced tomato<br>2 tbsp crumbled feta cheese<br>2 tbsp Greek dressing | cup<br>Brown rice: 1/2 cup | pineappl e, and coconut water |

| 35 | Greek yogurt: 1/2 cup<br>Berries: 1/4 cup<br>Chia seeds: 1 tbsp | Turkey and vegetable stir-fry: 4 oz sliced turkey breast<br>1 cup mixed vegetables<br>1/2 cup cooked brown rice | Baked salmon: 6 oz<br>Roasted Brussels sprouts: 1 cup | Mixed nuts: 1/4 cup<br>Cucumber: 1/2 cup<br>Hummus: 2 tbsp |

## WEEK 6

| Day | Breakfast | Lunch | Dinner | Snacks |
| --- | --- | --- | --- | --- |
| 36 | Whole grain | Chicken Caesar | Grilled steak: 6 | Rice cakes: |

| | | | | |
|---|---|---|---|---|
| | toast: 1 slice<br>Mashed avocado: 1/2 avocado<br>Poached egg: 1 | salad: 4 oz grilled chicken breast<br>2 cups romaine lettuce<br>1/4 cup whole grain croutons<br>2 tbsp Caesar dressing | oz<br>Mixed roasted vegetables: 1 cup | 2<br>Almond butter: 2 tbsp<br>Apple slices: 1 medium<br>Greek yogurt: 1/2 cup |
| 37 | Chia seed pudding: 1/2 cup<br>Berries: 1/4 cup | Lentil soup: 1 cup<br>Mixed greens salad: 2 cups<br> | Turkey chili: 1 cup<br>Mixed vegetables: 1/2 cup | Carrot sticks: 1/2 cup<br>Greek yogurt: 1/2 |

| | | | | |
|---|---|---|---|---|
| | | 1/4 cup lentils<br>1/4 cup diced cucumbe r<br>1/4 cup diced tomato<br>2 tbsp vinaigrett e | | cup<br>Honey: 1 tbsp |
| 38 | Whole grain waffles: 2<br>Al mond butter: 2 tbsp<br>Sliced strawberr ies: 1/2 | Grilled chicken salad: 4 oz grilled chicken breast<b r>2 cups mixed greens<br>1/4 | Baked tilapia: 6 oz<br>R oasted asparagu s: 1 cup<br>Cooked quinoa: 1/2 cup | Rice cakes: 2<br>Al mond butter: 2 tbsp<br>Sliced bell peppers: 1/2 |

|  |  |  |  |  |
| --- | --- | --- | --- | --- |
|  | cup | cup<br>diced cucumbe r<br>1/4 cup diced tomato<br>2 tbsp balsamic vinaigrett e |  | cup<br>Guacam ole: 2 tbsp |
| 39 | 2 scramble d eggs<br>1 cup spinach<br>1 slice whole grain toast | Lentil soup: 1 cup<br>Mixed greens salad: 2 cups<br>1/4 cup lentils<br>1/4 cup diced | Grilled chicken breast: 6 oz<br>Mi xed roasted vegetabl es: 1 cup<br>1/2 cup cooked | Carrot sticks: 1 medium<br>Gree k yogurt: 1/2 cup<br>Almonds: 2 tbsp |

| | | | | |
|---|---|---|---|---|
| | | tomato<br>1/4 cup diced cucumbe r<br>2 tbsp vinaigrett e | quinoa | |
| 40 | 1 cup oats<br>1/2 sliced banana<br>1 tbsp chopped walnuts | Turkey and avocado wrap: 4 oz sliced turkey breast<br>1/4 avocado<br>1 whole grain tortilla<br>1/2 cup | Baked cod: 6 oz<br>Quinoa: 1/2 cup<br>Steamed broccoli: 1 cup | Apple slices: 1 medium<br>Peanut butter: 2 tbsp<br>Cottage cheese: 1/2 cup<br>Pineappl e chunks: |

| | | mixed greens | | 1/2 cup |
| 41 | Smoothie: 1 cup spinach<br>1/2 banana<br>1/2 cup almond milk<br>1 scoop protein powder | Greek salad with grilled chicken: 4 oz grilled chicken breast<br>1/2 cup mixed greens<br>1/4 cup diced cucumber<br>1/4 cup diced tomato< | Stir-fried tofu: 4 oz<br>Mixed vegetables: 1 cup<br>Brown rice: 1/2 cup | Edamame: 1/2 cup<br>Smoothie: 1 cup spinach, pineapple, and coconut water |

|  |  |  |  |  |
| --- | --- | --- | --- | --- |
|  |  | br>2 tbsp crumbled feta cheese<br>2 tbsp Greek dressing |  |  |
| 42 | Greek yogurt: 1/2 cup<br>Berries: 1/4 cup<br>Chia seeds: 1 tbsp | Turkey and vegetable stir-fry: 4 oz sliced turkey breast<br>1 cup mixed vegetables<br>1/2 cup cooked | Baked salmon: 6 oz<br>Roasted Brussels sprouts: 1 cup | Mixed nuts: 1/4 cup<br>Cucumber: 1/2 cup<br>Hummus: 2 tbsp |

| | | | | |
|---|---|---|---|---|
| | | brown rice | | |

## WEEK 7

| Day | Breakfast | Lunch | Dinner | Snacks |
|---|---|---|---|---|
| 43 | Whole grain toast: 1 slice<br>Mashed avocado: 1/2 avocado<br>Poached egg: 1 | Chicken Caesar salad: 4 oz grilled chicken breast<br>2 cups romaine lettuce<br>1/4 cup whole grain croutons<br>2 tbsp | Grilled steak: 6 oz<br>Mixed roasted vegetables: 1 cup | Rice cakes: 2<br>Almond butter: 2 tbsp<br>Apple slices: 1 medium<br>Greek yogurt: 1/2 cup |

| | | Caesar dressing | | |
|---|---|---|---|---|
| 44 | Chia seed pudding: 1/2 cup<br>Berries: 1/4 cup | Lentil soup: 1 cup<br>Mixed greens salad: 2 cups<br>1/4 cup lentils<br>1/4 cup diced cucumber<br>1/4 cup diced tomato<br>2 tbsp vinaigrette | Turkey chili: 1 cup<br>Mixed vegetables: 1/2 cup | Carrot sticks: 1/2 cup<br>Greek yogurt: 1/2 cup<br>Honey: 1 tbsp |
| 45 | Whole | Grilled | Baked | Rice |

| | | | |
|---|---|---|---|
| | grain waffles: 2<br>Almond butter: 2 tbsp<br>Sliced strawberries: 1/2 cup | chicken salad: 4 oz grilled chicken breast<br>2 cups mixed greens<br>1/4 cup diced cucumber<br>1/4 cup diced tomato<br>2 tbsp balsamic vinaigrette | tilapia: 6 oz<br>Roasted asparagus: 1 cup<br>Cooked quinoa: 1/2 cup | cakes: 2<br>Almond butter: 2 tbsp<br>Sliced bell peppers: 1/2 cup<br>Guacamole: 2 tbsp |
| 46 | Scrambled eggs | Lentil soup: 1 | Grilled chicken | Carrot sticks: 1 |

|  | with spinach and mushrooms<br>1 slice whole grain toast | cup<br>Mixed greens salad: 2 cups<br>1/4 cup lentils<br>1/4 cup diced tomato<br>1/4 cup diced cucumber<br>2 tbsp vinaigrette | breast: 6 oz<br>Mixed roasted vegetables: 1 cup<br>1/2 cup cooked quinoa | medium<br>Greek yogurt: 1/2 cup<br>Almonds: 2 tbsp |
|---|---|---|---|---|
| 47 | Oatmeal topped with sliced bananas | Turkey and avocado wrap: 4 oz sliced | Baked cod: 6 oz<br>Quinoa: 1/2 | Apple slices: 1 medium<br>Peanut butter: |

|  |  |  |  |  |
| --- | --- | --- | --- | --- |
|  | and walnuts | turkey breast<br>1/4 avocado<br>1 whole grain tortilla<br>1/2 cup mixed greens | cup<br>Steamed broccoli: 1 cup | 2 tbsp<br>Cottage cheese: 1/2 cup<br>Pineapple chunks: 1/2 cup |
| 48 | Smoothie: 1 cup spinach<br>1/2 banana<br>1/2 cup almond milk<br>1 scoop protein powder | Greek salad with grilled chicken: 4 oz grilled chicken breast<br>1/2 cup mixed | Stir-fried tofu: 4 oz<br>Mixed vegetables: 1 cup<br>Brown rice: 1/2 cup | Edamame: 1/2 cup<br>Smoothie: 1 cup spinach, pineapple, and coconut water |

| | | greens<br>1/4 cup diced cucumbe r<br>1/4 cup diced tomato<br>2 tbsp crumbled feta cheese<br>2 tbsp Greek dressing | | |
|---|---|---|---|---|
| 49 | Greek yogurt: 1/2 cup<br>Berries: | Turkey and vegetabl e stir-fry: 4 oz | Baked salmon: 6 oz<br>R oasted | Mixed nuts: 1/4 cup<br> Cucumb er: 1/2 |

| | 1/4 cup<br>Chia seeds: 1 tbsp | sliced turkey breast<br>1 cup mixed vegetabl es<br>1/ 2 cup cooked brown rice | Brussels sprouts: 1 cup | cup<br>Hummus : 2 tbsp |

**WEEK 8**

| Day | Breakfas t | Lunch | Dinner | Snacks |
| --- | --- | --- | --- | --- |
| 50 | Whole grain toast: 1 slice<br>Mashed avocado: 1/2 avocado | Chicken Caesar salad: 4 oz grilled chicken breast<b r>2 cups romaine | Grilled steak: 6 oz<br>Mi xed roasted vegetabl es: 1 cup | Rice cakes: 2<br>Al mond butter: 2 tbsp<br>Apple slices: 1 |

| | | | | |
|---|---|---|---|---|
| | <br>Poached egg: 1 | lettuce<br>1/4 cup whole grain croutons<br>2 tbsp Caesar dressing | | medium<br>Greek yogurt: 1/2 cup |
| 51 | Chia seed pudding: 1/2 cup<br>Berries: 1/4 cup | Lentil soup: 1 cup<br>Mixed greens salad: 2 cups<br>1/4 cup lentils<br>1/4 cup diced cucumber<br>1/4 | Turkey chili: 1 cup<br>Mixed vegetables: 1/2 cup | Carrot sticks: 1/2 cup<br>Greek yogurt: 1/2 cup<br>Honey: 1 tbsp |

| | | | | |
|---|---|---|---|---|
| | | cup diced tomato<br>2 tbsp vinaigrette | | |
| 52 | Whole grain waffles: 2<br>Almond butter: 2 tbsp<br>Sliced strawberries: 1/2 cup | Grilled chicken salad: 4 oz grilled chicken breast<br>2 cups mixed greens<br>1/4 cup diced cucumber<br>1/4 cup diced | Baked tilapia: 6 oz<br>Roasted asparagus: 1 cup<br>Cooked quinoa: 1/2 cup | Rice cakes: 2<br>Almond butter: 2 tbsp<br>Sliced bell peppers: 1/2 cup<br>Guacamole: 2 tbsp |

| | | tomato<br>2 tbsp balsamic vinaigrette | | |
|---|---|---|---|---|
| 53 | Scrambled eggs with spinach and mushrooms<br>1 slice whole grain toast | Lentil soup: 1 cup<br>Mixed greens salad: 2 cups<br>1/4 cup lentils<br>1/4 cup diced tomato<br>1/4 cup diced cucumber<br>2 | Grilled chicken breast: 6 oz<br>Mixed roasted vegetables: 1 cup<br>1/2 cup cooked quinoa | Carrot sticks: 1 medium<br>Greek yogurt: 1/2 cup<br>Almonds: 2 tbsp |

| | | tbsp vinaigrette | | |
|---|---|---|---|---|
| 54 | Oatmeal topped with sliced bananas and walnuts | Turkey and avocado wrap: 4 oz sliced turkey breast<br>1/4 avocado<br>1 whole grain tortilla<br>1/2 cup mixed greens | Baked cod: 6 oz<br>Quinoa: 1/2 cup<br>Steamed broccoli: 1 cup | Apple slices: 1 medium<br>Peanut butter: 2 tbsp<br>Cottage cheese: 1/2 cup<br>Pineapple chunks: 1/2 cup |
| 55 | Smoothie: 1 cup spinach<br>1/2 | Greek salad with grilled | Stir-fried tofu: 4 oz<br>Mixed | Edamame: 1/2 cup<br>Smoothi |

banana<br>1/2 cup almond milk<br>1 scoop protein powder

chicken: 4 oz grilled chicken breast<br>1/2 cup mixed greens<br>1/4 cup diced cucumber<br>1/4 cup diced tomato<br>2 tbsp crumbled feta cheese<br>2 tbsp

vegetables: 1 cup<br>Brown rice: 1/2 cup

e: 1 cup spinach, pineapple, and coconut water

| Day | Breakfast | Lunch | Dinner | Snacks |
|---|---|---|---|---|
| | | Greek dressing | | |
| 56 | Greek yogurt: 1/2 cup<br>Berries: 1/4 cup<br>Chia seeds: 1 tbsp | Turkey and vegetable stir-fry: 4 oz sliced turkey breast<br>1 cup mixed vegetables<br>1/2 cup cooked brown rice | Baked salmon: 6 oz<br>Roasted Brussels sprouts: 1 cup | Mixed nuts: 1/4 cup<br>Cucumber: 1/2 cup<br>Hummus: 2 tbsp |

**WEEK 9**

| Day | Breakfast | Lunch | Dinner | Snacks |
|---|---|---|---|---|

| 57 | Whole grain toast: 1 slice<br>Mashed avocado: 1/2 avocado<br>Poached egg: 1 | Chicken Caesar salad: 4 oz grilled chicken breast<br>2 cups romaine lettuce<br>1/4 cup whole grain croutons<br>2 tbsp Caesar dressing | Grilled steak: 6 oz<br>Mixed roasted vegetables: 1 cup | Rice cakes: 2<br>Almond butter: 2 tbsp<br>Apple slices: 1 medium<br>Greek yogurt: 1/ |
|---|---|---|---|---|
| 58 | 1 cup oats<br>1/2 sliced banana< | 1 cup lentil soup<br>2 cups mixed | 4 turkey meatballs<br>1 cup zucchini | 1 medium apple<br>2 tbsp peanut |

| | | | | |
|---|---|---|---|---|
| | br>1 tbsp walnuts | greens< br>2 tbsp vinaigrett e | noodles< br>1/2 cup marinara sauce | butter<br >1/2 cup cottage cheese< br>1/2 cup pineappl e chunks |
| 59 | 2 scramble d eggs<br >1 cup spinach< br>1/2 cup cherry tomatoes <br>1 slice whole grain toast | 4 oz grilled chicken breast<b r>2 cups mixed greens< br>1/2 cucumbe r<br>1/2 bell pepper< br>2 tbsp balsamic | 4 oz baked salmon< br>1 cup roasted asparagu s<br>1/2 cup cooked quinoa | 1 medium carrot<br >2 tbsp hummus <br>1/2 cup Greek yogurt<b r>1 tbsp almonds |

| | | vinaigrett<br>e | | |
| --- | --- | --- | --- | --- |
| 60 | 1 cup spinach<br>1/2 banana<br>1/2 cup almond milk<br>1 scoop protein powder | 4 oz grilled chicken breast<br>2 cups romaine lettuce<br>2 tbsp Caesar dressing | 6 grilled shrimp<br>1/2 cup cooked brown rice<br>1 cup steamed broccoli | 1/4 cup mixed nuts<br>1 cup whole grain cereal<br>1/2 cup skim milk |

# MEAL PREP TIPS

Meal prep is a crucial aspect of a successful weight loss journey, especially when aiming to lose a significant amount of weight like 40kg in two months. Here are some meal prep tips tailored to this ambitious goal:

1. **Plan Ahead:** Take time to plan your meals for the week, considering your calorie and nutrient needs for weight loss. Choose

recipes that are balanced, nutritious, and aligned with your dietary preferences and goals.

2. **Batch Cooking:** Dedicate a day or two each week to batch cooking large quantities of healthy meals and portioning them out into individual servings. This allows you to have ready-made meals on hand for busy days when cooking from scratch isn't feasible.

3. **Focus on Whole Foods:** Prioritize whole, minimally processed foods in your meal prep, such as lean proteins, fruits, vegetables, whole grains, and healthy fats. These foods provide essential nutrients and support satiety, making it easier to stick to your calorie goals.

4. **Portion Control:** Use portion control tools like measuring cups, food scales, or pre-portioned containers to ensure that each meal aligns with your calorie and portion size goals. This helps prevent overeating and promotes mindful eating habits.

5. **Include Variety:** Keep your meals interesting and satisfying by incorporating a variety of flavors, textures, and cuisines into

your meal prep. Experiment with different recipes, ingredients, and cooking methods to prevent boredom and promote adherence to your weight loss plan.

6. **Prep Snacks and Grab-and-Go Options:** Prepare healthy snacks and grab-and-go options to have on hand for when hunger strikes between meals. Opt for nutrient-rich snacks like fruit, nuts, yogurt, or cut-up vegetables with hummus to satisfy cravings and keep you on track with your weight loss goals.

7. **Store Properly:** Store your prepped meals and snacks in airtight containers in the refrigerator or freezer to maintain freshness and prevent spoilage. Label containers with the date and contents to facilitate identification.

8. **Stay Flexible:** While meal prep can save time and simplify healthy eating, it's important to stay flexible and adapt to changes in your schedule or preferences. Allow for some wiggle room in your meal plan to accommodate spontaneous events or cravings without derailing your progress.

By implementing these meal prep tips, you can set yourself up for success in your weight loss journey and work towards your goal of losing 40kg in two months. Remember to stay consistent, stay focused on your goals, and celebrate your progress along the way!

# BUILDING BALANCED MEALS

Building balanced meals is essential for supporting weight loss. Here's a brief overview of how to create balanced meals:

1. **Include Lean Protein:** Start by incorporating a lean source of protein into each meal. This could be chicken breast, fish, tofu, beans, or lentils. Protein promotes satiety, maintains muscular mass, and aids metabolism.

2. **Add Fiber-Rich Carbohydrates**: Include complex carbohydrates that are high in fiber, such as whole grains (brown rice,quinoa), fruits, and vegetables. Fiber helps to control blood sugar levels, promotes fullness, and improves digestive health.

3. **Incorporate Healthy Fats:** Include healthy fat sources in your meals, such as nuts, seeds, olive oil, and fatty fish like salmon. Healthy fats provide essential nutrients, support hormone production, and enhance the absorption of fat-soluble vitamins.

4. **Include Plenty of Vegetables:** Make vegetables a central part of your meals, aiming to fill half of your plate with non-starchy vegetables like leafy greens,

and carrots. Vegetables are low in calories and high in nutrients, helping to bulk up meals without adding excess calories.

5. **Mind Your Portions:** Pay attention to portion sizes to avoid overeating and ensure that your meals are balanced in terms of calories and nutrients. Use visual cues, measuring tools, or pre-portioned containers to help you control portion sizes and prevent mindless eating.

6. **Stay Hydrated:** Don't forget to include fluids as part of your meal planning. Water is essential for overall health and can help support weight loss by promoting hydration and reducing calorie intake from sugary beverages.

# CHAPTER 4: ADAPTING TO CHALLENGES

When navigating changes in your weight loss journey, remain flexible with your approach. Adjust your meal plan, exercise routine, and mindset to overcome plateaus or setbacks

## OVERCOMING PLATEAUS

Overcoming plateaus in weight loss requires persistence and strategic adjustments. Here's how to break through:

1. **Review Your Habits**: Reflect on your eating and exercise habits. Are there areas where you could improve consistency or intensity?

2. **Adjust Your Caloric Intake**: Re-evaluate your calorie intake. As you lose weight, your body may require fewer calories to maintain progress.

3. **Mix Up Your Workouts**: Add variation to your training program. Try new activities or increase the intensity to challenge your body in different ways.

4. **Focus on Strength Training:** Build lean muscle mass through strength training.

Muscle burns more calories at rest, aiding in weight loss.

5. **Prioritize Sleep and Stress Management:** Get enough sleep and manage your stress levels. Poor sleep and excessive stress levels can impede weight loss efforts.

6. **Stay Hydrated**: Drink plenty of water. Dehydration can impact metabolism and energy levels.

7. **Be Patient and Consistent**: Plateaus are normal. Maintain your commitment to your goals and place your trust in the process. Consistency is key to long-term success.

By making strategic adjustments to your routine and staying patient and consistent, you can overcome plateaus and continue progressing towards your weight loss goals.

# DINING OUT STRATEGIES

Navigating dining out while on a weight loss journey can present challenges, but with the right strategies, it's possible to enjoy restaurant meals while staying on track with your goals.

Here are some tips for dining out:

**Plan Ahead:**

Check the restaurant's menu online in advance to review your options and make healthier choices.
Look for dishes that are grilled, steamed, or roasted, and avoid items that are fried, breaded, or creamy.

**Control Portions**:
Be mindful of portion sizes, which are often larger than necessary. Consider splitting an entrée with a dining companion or requesting a half serving. Opt for appetizers or starters as your main course, or request a to-go box upfront to save half of your meal for later.

**Choose Wisely:**
Prioritize lean protein sources such as grilled chicken, fish, or tofu, and load up on vegetables as side dishes or main courses.
Avoid heavy sauces, dressings, and toppings, and ask for them on the side so you can control the amount you use.

**Customize Your Order:**
Don't hesitate to ask for substitutions or modifications to fit your dietary preferences and needs. For example, request steamed vegetables instead of fries or a salad instead of rice.

**Be Mindful of Beverages:**
Opt for water, unsweetened tea, or other calorie-free beverages instead of sugary sodas,

cocktails, or alcoholic drinks, which can add unnecessary calories.

If you choose to drink alcohol, do so in moderation and be aware of its impact on your calorie intake.

**Practice Portion Control:**

Use visual cues to estimate portion sizes. For example, a serving of meat should be about the size of a deck of cards, and a serving of grains should be about the size of a tennis ball.Consider ordering an appetizer or splitting an entrée with a friend to avoid overeating.

**Listen to Your Body:**

Pay close attention to your hunger and fullness signs during the meal. Stop eating when you are content, not when your plate is empty.

Take your time and savor each bite, enjoying the flavors and textures of your meal.

**Practice Moderation:**

It's okay to indulge occasionally, but aim to make healthier choices most of the time. If you do splurge on a high-calorie meal, balance it out with lighter options for your other meals that day.

By implementing these dining out strategies, you can enjoy restaurant meals without derailing your weight loss progress. Remember that consistency and moderation are key, and focus on making mindful choices that align with your goals.

# CHAPTER 5: INCORPORATE PHYSICAL ACTIVITY

Incorporating physical activity into your weight loss journey is an essential component for achieving significant results in a relatively short period. Here's how to gracefully integrate exercise into your two-month weight loss plan:

Set Realistic Goals

Find Activities You Enjoy: Whether it's dancing, swimming, hiking, cycling, or practicing yoga, selecting activities that you genuinely enjoy will increase your likelihood of sticking with them long-term.

Aim for a well-rounded exercise routine that incorporates cardiovascular, strength training, flexibility, and balance exercises. Mixing up your workouts not only prevents boredom but also ensures that you're targeting different muscle groups and enhancing overall fitness levels.

Start Slowly and Progress Gradually: If you're new to exercise or returning after a hiatus, start with low-impact activities and gradually increase intensity and duration over time. Listen to your body's cues and avoid pushing yourself too hard, especially in the beginning stages of your fitness journey.

Schedule Regular Workouts: Treat exercise as an essential part of your daily routine by scheduling dedicated workout sessions into your calendar. Consistency is key to seeing results, so aim for at least 30 minutes of moderate-intensity exercise most days of the week.

Life can be unpredictable, and sticking to a rigid exercise schedule isn't always feasible. Be flexible and adaptable by embracing opportunities to move whenever and wherever you can, whether it's taking the stairs, walking during phone calls, or doing quick workouts at home.

Pay attention to how your body reacts to exercise and tailor your routines accordingly. If you're feeling fatigued or experiencing discomfort, give yourself permission to rest and recover. Remember that rest days are just as important as active days in preventing burnout and injury.

Celebrate Your Progress: Celebrate your achievements, no matter how small they may seem. Whether it's reaching a fitness milestone, mastering a new exercise, or simply feeling stronger and more energized, acknowledge and celebrate your progress along the way.Incorporating physical activity into your weight loss journey is not only beneficial for burning calories and shedding pounds but also for improving overall health, boosting mood, and enhancing quality of life. Approach exercise with grace, patience, and positivity, and you'll be amazed at the transformation you can achieve in just two months.

# BALANCING EXERCISES WITH NUTRITION

Balancing exercise with nutrition is essential for achieving optimal health and maximizing results in your weight loss journey. Here's how to effectively harmonize these two components:

**Fuel Your Workouts**: Prioritize consuming a balanced meal or snack containing carbohydrates, protein, and healthy fats before and after your workouts to support energy levels, muscle repair, and recovery.

**Hydrate Adequately:** Drink plenty of water throughout the day, especially before, during, and after exercise, to replenish fluids lost through sweat and maintain proper hydration levels.

**Timing Matters**: Pay attention to the timing of your meals and snacks in relation to your workouts. Aim to eat a balanced meal or snack containing carbohydrates and protein 1-3 hours before exercising to provide sustained energy and support muscle function. After your workout, refuel with a combination of carbohydrates and protein to aid in muscle recovery and replenish glycogen stores.

**Quality Over Quantity:** Focus on consuming nutrient-dense foods that provide essential vitamins, minerals, and antioxidants to support overall health and well-being. Choose whole, minimally processed foods such as fruits, vegetables, lean proteins, whole grains, and healthy fats to nourish your body and optimize exercise performance.

**Match Nutrition to Activity Level**: Adjust your calorie intake and macronutrient distribution based on your activity level and fitness goals. If you're engaging in intense or prolonged exercise sessions, you may need to increase your calorie and carbohydrate intake to fuel performance and support recovery. On rest days or during periods of lighter activity, adjust your nutrition accordingly to match your energy needs.

**Seek professional guidance**

By balancing exercise with nutrition, you can optimize your performance, enhance recovery, and achieve sustainable results in your weight loss journey. Prioritize nourishing your body with nutrient-rich foods that support your energy needs and promote overall health and well-being.

# CHAPTER 6: IDEAL EXERCISE PLAN TO INCORPORATE WITH THE MEAL PLAN FOR ONE MONTH

Here's a one-month exercise plan designed to promote drastic weight loss:

**Week 1**

**Cardiovascular Focus**

Day 1-3: Walking

Duration: 30 minutes
Description: Start with brisk walking sessions. Focus on maintaining a steady pace, swinging your arms, and engaging your core muscles. Slowly increase your speed as you become more comfortable.

Click to view an effective description of how to walk for exercise.

Day 4: Rest

Description: Rest is essential for recovery and muscle repair. Use this day to relax and rejuvenate.

Duration: 20-25 minutes
Description: Begin with a light jog, gradually increasing your pace as you warm up. Focus on proper form, landing softly on your feet, and breathing rhythmically. Alternate between jogging and walking if needed.

Click to watch an effective description of how to jog.

Click to watch an effective description of how to jog.


Week 2
## Strength Training

Day 8-10: Bodyweight Exercises

Exercises: Push-ups, squats, lunges, planks
Sets/Reps: 3 sets of 10-12 reps for each exercise
Description: Perform each exercise with proper form, focusing on controlled movements and engaging the targeted muscles. Take short breaks between sets to catch your breath.

Click to watch an effective description of how to plank.
Click to watch an effective description of how to push-ups.

Click to watch an effective description of how to squat.
Click to watch an effective description of how to lunges.

## Day 11: Rest

Description: Allow your muscles to recover and repair from the previous workouts.

## Day 12-14: Resistance Band Workout

Exercises: Banded squats, banded rows, banded chest press, banded lateral walks
Sets/Reps: 3 sets of 12-15 reps for each exercise
Description: Use resistance bands to add intensity to your workouts. Focus on maintaining tension throughout each movement and controlling the resistance.

Click to watch an effective description of how to squat using a band.
Click to watch an effective description of how to chest press using a band.
Click to watch an effective description of how to take lateral walks using a band.
Click to watch an effective description of how to undertake banded rows.

Week 3

## Interval Training



Exercises: Jumping jacks, mountain climbers, burpees, high knees
Duration: 20-25 minutes (including warm-up and cool-down)
Description: Alternate between short bursts of high-intensity exercise and periods of rest or low-intensity recovery. Push yourself during the work intervals, aiming for maximum effort.

Click to watch an effective description of how to undertake HIIT for weight loss.

Click to watch an effective description of how to undertake HIIT for weight loss.

Day 18: Rest

Description: Take a day off to allow your body to recover and prepare for the next phase of training.

Day 19-21: Circuit Training

Exercises: Full-body circuit (e.g., jumping squats, push-ups, lunges, plank)

Sets/Reps: Perform each exercise for 30 seconds, followed by 15 seconds of rest. Complete 3-4 rounds.

Description: Move through each exercise in the circuit without rest between movements. Focus on maintaining good form and intensity throughout the workout.



**Active Recovery and Flexibility**



Duration: 30-45 minutes

Description: Focus on gentle, flowing movements that improve flexibility, mobility, and balance. Pay attention to your breath and follow your body's cues.

Click to watch an effective description of how to undertake yoga.

Click to watch an effective description of how to undertake yoga.

Click to watch an effective description of how to undertake pilates.



Description: Take a day to rest or engage in light, low-impact activities such as walking or swimming to promote recovery.

Duration: 15-20 minutes
Description: Perform a series of stretches targeting major muscle groups, focusing on lengthening and releasing tension. Hold each stretch for 20-30 seconds, taking care not to bounce.

Click to watch an effective description of how to undertake stretches.

Remember to consult with a healthcare professional before starting any new exercise program, especially if you have any underlying health conditions or concerns.

# TRACKING PROGRESS

One essential tool that can significantly impact your success is the process of tracking. Whether you're aiming to shed a few pounds or undergo a drastic transformation, monitoring your progress through tracking can provide invaluable insights, accountability, and motivation along the way.
Tracking goes beyond simply recording numbers on a scale or calories consumed; it's about cultivating

mindfulness, awareness, and self-reflection throughout your weight loss journey. By tracking your efforts and results, you can identify patterns, celebrate successes, and identify areas for improvement, guiding you towards sustainable lifestyle changes and long-term success, remember that tracking is not about perfection but progress. Embrace the process with curiosity, compassion, and resilience, and trust that every step you take towards self-awareness and improvement brings you closer to the healthier, happier version of yourself you aspire to be.

## MONITORING WEIGHT LOSS

Weigh yourself using a reliable scale and record your weight in a journal or app. Track trends over time rather than focusing on daily fluctuations. Additionally, monitor other indicators of progress such as changes in body measurements, energy levels, and how your clothes fit.

Celebrate your successes, learn from setbacks, and adjust your approach as needed to continue moving towards your weight loss goals with confidence and determination.

# ASSESSING BODY MEASUREMENTS

Start by measuring key areas such as your waist, hips, chest, arms, and thighs using a flexible measuring tape. Record these measurements regularly, such as once a week or once a month, to track changes over time. While the scale may not always reflect your progress accurately, changes in body measurements can provide a more comprehensive picture of your body transformation. Look for trends and improvements in inches lost rather than focusing solely on the numbers. Celebrate your achievements and use body measurements as a motivating tool to stay committed to your weight loss journey.

# CELEBRATING ACHIEVEMENTS

Celebrating achievements along your weight loss journey is essential for maintaining motivation and reinforcing positive behaviors.
Whether you've reached a significant milestone or achieved a small victory, taking the time to celebrate your accomplishments can boost your morale and propel you forward towards your goals. Here are some ways to celebrate your weight loss achievements:

- **Acknowledge Progress**: Take a moment to reflect on how far you've come since starting your weight loss journey. Celebrate the progress you've made, whether it's losing a certain number of pounds, fitting into smaller clothes, or improving your fitness levels.

- **Reward Yourself:** Treat yourself to a non-food reward as a symbol of your hard work and dedication. This could be anything from buying new workout clothes or shoes to indulging in a spa day or booking a weekend getaway

- **Share Your Success:** Share your achievements with friends, family, or a support group who can celebrate with you. Sharing your successes not only reinforces your commitment but also inspires others on their own weight loss journeys.

- **Create Milestone Rewards:** Set up milestone rewards for reaching specific weight loss goals. For example, treat yourself to a massage, a new book, or a day trip when you hit a certain milestone.

- **Document Your Journey:** Keep a journal or scrapbook documenting your weight loss journey, including progress photos, motivational quotes, and personal reflections. Reviewing how far you've come can be a powerful reminder of your achievements and inspire you to keep pushing forward.

- **Celebrate Non-Scale Victories:** Recognize and celebrate non-scale victories such as improved energy levels, better sleep, increased confidence, and improved overall health. These achievements are just as important as the number on the scale and deserve to be celebrated.

- **Plan a Celebration Meal:** Enjoy a special meal or treat yourself to your favorite healthy dish to celebrate reaching a milestone.

Just be mindful of portion sizes and choose nutritious options that align with your weight loss goals.

Remember that celebrating achievements is not only about rewarding yourself but also about acknowledging your hard work, dedication, and commitment to your health and well-being. By celebrating your successes along the way, you'll stay motivated, inspired, and empowered to continue making progress towards your weight loss goals.

# CHAPTER 7: MAINTENANCE AND LONG TERM SUCCESS

After achieving your desired weight loss goals, transitioning into a maintenance phase is essential for sustaining your progress and preventing regain. Here's how to approach maintenance and ensure long-term success:

- **Establish Sustainable Habits:** Focus on adopting healthy lifestyle habits that you can maintain for the long term. This includes eating a balanced diet, staying active, managing stress, prioritizing sleep, and practicing self-care.

- **Monitor Your Progress:** Continue to monitor your weight and body measurements regularly, even after reaching your initial goals. This allows you to catch any changes early and make adjustments as needed to stay on track.

- **Stay Active:** Maintain a regular exercise routine that includes a combination of cardiovascular, strength training, and flexibility exercises. Aim for at least 150 minutes of moderate-intensity aerobic activity or 75 minutes of vigorous-intensity activity each week, along with muscle-strengthening activities on two or more days per week.

- Mindful Eating: Practice mindful eating by paying attention to hunger and fullness cues, eating slowly, and savoring your food. Be mindful of portion sizes and choose nutrient-dense foods that nourish your body and support your overall health.

- Stay Accountable: Continue to hold yourself accountable to your goals by tracking your food intake, exercise, and progress. Consider joining a support group, working with a coach, or partnering with a friend for added accountability and motivation.

- Adapt to Challenges: Be prepared to face challenges along the way, such as holidays, vacations, or periods of stress. Instead of viewing setbacks as failures, see them as opportunities to learn and grow. Develop strategies for managing triggers and staying on track during challenging times.

- Seek Support: Surround yourself with a supporting network of friends, family, or experts who can provide the mental, emotional and physical support you require.

- Encouragement, advice, and guidance as needed. Lean on your support system during difficult times and celebrate your successes together.

# STRATEGIES FOR WEIGHT MAINTENANCE

Maintaining weight loss requires a strategic approach to ensure long-term success. Here are some helpful ways for maintaining your weight::

- **Monitor Your Weight:** Continue to weigh yourself regularly, whether it's daily, weekly, or monthly. This helps you stay aware of any changes and allows you to address them promptly if needed.

- **Stay Active:** Maintain a regular exercise routine that includes a combination of cardiovascular, strength training, and flexibility exercises. Aim for 150 minutes of moderate-intensity aerobic activity or 75 minutes of vigorous-intensity activity per week, with muscle-strengthening activities on two or more days.

- **Practice Portion Control:** Practice Portion Control: Pay attention to your body's hunger and fullness signs. Focus on filling your plate with nutrient-dense foods like fruits, vegetables, lean proteins, and whole grains.

- **Eat Mindfully:** Practice mindful eating by paying attention to your food choices, eating slowly, and savoring each bite. Avoid distractions like television or smartphones while eating, and focus on enjoying the flavors and textures of your food.

- **Balance Your Diet:** Continue to prioritize a balanced diet that includes a variety of nutrient-rich foods from all food groups. Aim to consume plenty of fruits, vegetables, lean proteins, whole grains, and healthy fats to support your overall health and well-being.

- **Stay Hydrated:** Drink enough water throughout the day to keep your body hydrated and functioning properly.. Aim for at least eight 8-ounce glasses of water per day, and more if you're physically active or in hot weather.

- **Get Plenty of Sleep:** Prioritize adequate sleep each night, aiming for 7-9 hours for most adults. Lack of sleep can disrupt hormones that regulate hunger and appetite, leading to increased cravings and overeating.

- **Manage Stress:** Find healthy ways to manage stress, such as exercise, meditation, deep breathing exercises, or spending time with loved ones. Chronic stress can cause emotional eating and weight gain, therefore it's critical to develop good coping skills.

- **Stay Accountable:** Continue to hold yourself accountable to your weight loss goals by tracking your food intake, exercise, and progress. Consider joining a weight loss maintenance group or working with a coach to stay motivated and accountable.

- **Be Kind to Yourself:** Remember that maintaining weight loss is a journey, and there will be ups and downs along the way. Be kind to yourself and practice self-compassion, especially during challenging times. Focus on progress, not perfection, and celebrate your successes along the way.

By implementing these strategies for weight maintenance, you can increase your chances of long-term success and enjoy a healthy, balanced lifestyle for years to come. Remember that consistency is key, and small, sustainable changes over time can lead to lasting results.

# CONCLUSION

In conclusion, embarking on a weight loss journey is a transformative endeavor that requires dedication, commitment, and a willingness to embrace change. Throughout this book, we've explored the essential principles, strategies, and tools needed to achieve sustainable weight loss and create a healthier, happier lifestyle.

From setting realistic goals and adopting healthy habits to nourishing your body with nutritious foods and staying active, you have the power to take control of your health and transform your life. Remember that progress takes time, and every step you take towards your goals, no matter how small, brings you closer to success.

As you continue on your journey, stay focused on your reasons for wanting to change, draw strength from your achievements, and lean on your support system for encouragement and guidance. Celebrate your victories, learn from setbacks, and never lose sight of the incredible potential within you to create the life you desire.

With determination, perseverance, and a commitment to self-care, you have the power to achieve your weight loss goals and enjoy a lifetime of health, happiness, and vitality. Here's to your success, your well-being, and your journey towards a brighter, healthier future. You've got this!

# FINAL WORDS OF ENCOURAGEMENTS

As you close this book, remember: your journey is unique, and every step forward is a victory. Embrace the challenges, celebrate your successes, and stay true to yourself. You have the strength, resilience, and determination to achieve your goals. Keep believing in yourself, stay committed to your health, and know that you are capable of achieving anything you set your mind to. Your journey towards a healthier, happier you is just beginning. Go forth with confidence and embrace the incredible possibilities that lie ahead!

# ADDITIONAL RESOURCES FOR CONTINUED SUPPORT

Congratulations on completing this weight loss book! As you continue your journey towards a healthier lifestyle, we've compiled a list of additional resources and tools to support you along the way:

**Online Communities and Forums:**

Join online communities and forums dedicated to weight loss, nutrition, and fitness. Connect with others, share experiences, and find support from individuals on similar journeys.

Example: MyFitnessPal Community, Reddit's r/loseit, SparkPeople Community.

**Fitness and Nutrition Apps:**

Explore fitness and nutrition tracking apps to monitor your progress, set goals, and stay accountable. Many apps offer features such as meal planning, workout routines, and community support.

Example: MyFitnessPal, Lose It!, Fitbit, Nike Training Club.

**Books and Podcasts:**

Dive deeper into topics related to health, nutrition, fitness, and mindset by exploring books, podcasts, and audiobooks.

Example of Books: "The Obesity Code" by Dr. Jason Fung, "Atomic Habits" by James Clear, "The Whole30" by Melissa Hartwig Urban and Dallas Hartwig.

Example of Podcasts: "The Model Health Show" by Shawn Stevenson, "The Mind Pump Podcast" by Sal Di Stefano, Adam Schafer, and Justin Andrews.

**Professional Support:**

Consider seeking guidance from registered dietitians, nutritionists,
personal trainers, or therapists for personalized support and advice.

Example Of Organizations: Academy of Nutrition and Dietetics (AND), American Council on Exercise (ACE), National Strength and Conditioning Association (NSCA).

**Local Support Groups and Classes:**

Look for local weight loss support groups, wellness centers, or fitness classes in your community. Connecting with others face-to-face can provide additional motivation and accountability.

Example: Weight Watchers meetings, local gym classes, wellness workshops at community centers.

**Healthy Living Websites:**

Visit reputable websites dedicated to health, nutrition, and fitness for articles, recipes, workout routines, and tips.

Example of Websites: Healthline, Mayo Clinic, Verywell Fit, EatingWell.

**Wellness Events and Workshops:**

Attend wellness events, workshops, or seminars in your area to learn from experts, participate in interactive sessions, and connect with others.

Example: Health and wellness expos, cooking demonstrations, fitness retreats.

Remember to explore these resources and tools to find what works best for you. Stay committed to your goals, embrace the journey, and never hesitate to reach out for support when needed.

You have the power to transform your life and achieve lasting health and happiness. Best of luck on your continued journey towards a healthier, happier you!

# GROCERY SHOPPING LIST

Here's a comprehensive grocery shopping list to support your weight loss journey:

Proteins:

| | |
|---|---|
| Skinless chicken breast | Eggs |
| Lean ground turkey or chicken | Salmon or other fatty fish |
| Greek yogurt (plain, low fat or non fat) | Cottage cheese (low fat or non-fat) |
| Tofu or tempeh ( for vegetarian Options) | |

Vegetables:

| | |
|---|---|
| Leafy greens (spinach, kale, lettuce) | Bell peppers (assorted colors) |
| Broccoli | Cucumber |
| Cauliflower | Zucchini |
| Carrots | Tomatoes |

Fruits:

| | |
|---|---|
| Apples | Avocado |

| Bananas, Oranges | Grapefruit |
| --- | --- |
| Berries ( strawberries, blueberries, raspberries) | |

## Whole Grains:

| Quinoa | Brown rice |
| --- | --- |

## Oats (rolled or steel-cut):

| While wheat bread or wrapS | Whole grain pasta |
| --- | --- |

## Legumes:

| Black beans | Chick peas | Lentils |
| --- | --- | --- |

## Dairy and Dairy Alternatives:

| Low- fat or non-fat milk | Almond milk or other plant based milk |
| --- | --- |
| Low- fat cheese (mozzarella,feta) | Unsweetened Greek yogurt |

## Nuts and Seeds:

| Alomds | Walnuts | Chia seed | Flax seed |
| --- | --- | --- | --- |

## Healthy Fats:

| Olive oil | Coconut oil | Avocado oil |
| --- | --- | --- |

Herbs, Spices, and Condiments:

| Onion | Basil | Cumin | Paprika | Turmeric |
|---|---|---|---|---|
| Mustard | Low sodium soy sauce | | Balsamic | Oregano |

Miscellaneous:

| Mixed greens ( for salads) | Protein powder (optional) | Unsweetened applesauce |
|---|---|---|
| Sparking water | Herbal tea | Hummus |
| Whole grain crackers | Dark chocolate (70% or higher cocoa content) | |
| Vine ripened tomatoes | Unsweetened almond butter or peanut butter | |

Remember to check your pantry and fridge for items you may already have on hand before heading to the grocery store. Additionally, adjust quantities based on your preferences and meal plan. Happy shopping and happy cooking!

# COOKING TIPS AND TECHNIQUES

Here are some cooking tips and techniques to keep in mind when trying to shred fat

Choose Healthy Cooking Methods: Opt for cooking methods that use minimal added fat, such as baking, grilling, steaming, boiling, roasting, or sautéing with small amounts of olive oil or cooking spray. Avoid deep-frying or pan-frying foods, as these methods can add unnecessary calories and unhealthy fats.

Focus on Whole Foods: Base your meals around whole, minimally processed foods such as lean proteins, whole grains, fruits, and vegetables. These foods are naturally low in calories and high in nutrients, making them ideal choices for weight loss.

Portion Control: Pay attention to portion sizes when cooking and serving meals. Use measuring cups, spoons, or kitchen scales to portion out ingredients, especially high-calorie items like oils, nuts, and cheese. Fill half of your plate with veggies, one-fourth with lean protein, and the remaining quarter with whole grains or starchy vegetables.

Incorporate Flavorful Ingredients: Experiment with herbs, spices, citrus juices, and vinegar to add flavor to your meals without adding extra calories. Fresh herbs like basil, cilantro, and parsley can elevate the taste of dishes, while spices like garlic, cumin, and paprika add depth and complexity.

Bulk Up with Vegetables: Use vegetables as the star of your meals to add volume, fiber, and nutrients without a lot of calories. Incorporate vegetables into soups, stir-fries, casseroles, and salads to help you feel full and satisfied while reducing the calorie density of your meals.

Meal Prep: Spend some time each week prepping and portioning out ingredients to make healthy eating easier and more convenient. Cook batches of grains, proteins, and vegetables that can be used in multiple meals throughout the week. Portion out snacks and pre-cut fruits and vegetables for quick grab-and-go options.

Mindful Cooking: Practice mindfulness while cooking by focusing on the task at hand and paying attention to the flavors, textures, and aromas of the ingredients. To avoid mindless eating and overeating, turn off the television and smartphones while cooking.

Balanced Meals: Aim to create balanced meals that include a combination of lean protein, whole grains, healthy fats, and plenty of vegetables. This balance helps stabilize blood sugar levels, keep you feeling full longer, and provide a steady source of energy throughout the day.

By incorporating these cooking tips and techniques into your meal preparation routine, you can enjoy delicious, satisfying meals while supporting your weight loss goals.

# FREQUENTLY ASKED QUESTIONS

Here are 30 frequently asked questions about weight loss and their accurate answers:

**Q: How many calories should I consume to lose weight?**

A: The number of calories needed for weight loss varies based on factors such as age, gender, weight, height, activity level, and weight loss goals. In general, a calorie deficit of 500-1000 calories per day can result in 1-2 pounds of weight loss each week that is both safe and sustainable.

**Q: Can I lose weight without exercising?**

Yes, weight loss is primarily achieved through creating a calorie deficit, which can be accomplished through diet alone. However, incorporating exercise can enhance weight loss results, improve overall health, and support long-term weight maintenance.

**Q: How quickly can I expect to see results from my weight loss efforts?**

A: Weight loss results vary from person to person and depend on factors such as starting weight, calorie intake, physical activity level, and metabolism. While some individuals may see noticeable results within a few weeks, others may take longer to see changes.

**Q: Are certain foods or diets better for weight loss?**

A: There is no one-size-fits-all approach to weight loss, and different diets work for different people. However, focusing on whole, nutrient-dense foods such as fruits, vegetables, lean proteins, and whole grains can support weight loss and overall health.

**Q: How can I prevent weight regain after losing weight?**

A: To prevent weight regain, focus on adopting sustainable lifestyle habits such as regular exercise, mindful eating, portion control, and finding a healthy balance between nutrition and indulgence. Consistency, moderation, and self-awareness are key.

**Q: Is it feasible to remove fat from certain parts of the body?**

A: Spot reduction, or targeting fat loss in specific areas of the body, is a myth. While targeted exercises can strengthen and tone specific muscles, they do not reduce fat in that area. Instead, overall weight loss and body fat reduction occur through a combination of diet, exercise, and genetics.

Q: **Can I still eat my favourite meals while attempting to reduce weight?**
A: Yes, incorporating your favorite foods into your diet in moderation can help prevent feelings of deprivation and support long-term adherence to your weight loss plan. Focus on portion control, mindful eating, and balancing indulgences with nutrient-dense foods.

Q: **How can I keep motivated as I try to lose weight?**
A: Staying motivated during a weight loss journey can be challenging, but setting realistic goals, tracking progress, celebrating achievements, seeking support from friends or a support group, and focusing on the benefits of improved health and well-being can help maintain motivation.

Q: **Is it normal to experience weight fluctuations during a weight loss journey?**
A: Yes, weight fluctuations are normal and can occur due to factors such as water retention, menstrual cycle changes, digestion, and glycogen storage. Consider long-term patterns rather than daily changes on the scale.

Q: **How can I overcome weight loss plateaus?**
A: To overcome weight loss plateaus, consider adjusting your calorie intake, increasing physical

activity, varying your exercise routine, managing stress, ensuring adequate sleep, and reassessing your goals and strategies.

**Q: Can I have wine/alcohol while attempting to reduce weight?**

A: Alcohol contains calories and can contribute to weight gain if consumed in excess.Limiting alcohol intake and choosing lower-calorie options such as light beer, wine, or spirits mixed with calorie-free mixers can support weight loss efforts.

**Q: Do certain supplements or weight loss products help with weight loss?**

A: While some supplements or weight loss products may claim to aid in weight loss, their effectiveness and safety are often not supported by scientific evidence. It's best to focus on a balanced diet, regular exercise, and healthy lifestyle habits for sustainable weight loss.

**Q: How can I avoid bingeing or emotional eating?**

A: To avoid overeating or emotional eating, practice mindful eating, identify triggers for overeating, find alternative coping strategies for stress or emotions, and create a supportive environment that promotes healthy eating habits.

**Q: Is it safe to lose weight quickly?**

A: Rapid weight loss may result in nutrient deficiencies, muscle loss, and potential health risks.

A weight loss of 1-2 pounds per week is generally considered safe and sustainable for most individuals.

**Q: Can sleep affect weight loss?**
A: Yes, adequate sleep is important for weight loss and overall health. Lack of sleep can disrupt hormones thatregulate hunger and appetite,leading to increased cravings, overeating, and weight gain.

**Q: Should I avoid carbohydrates to lose weight?**
A: Carbohydrates are an essential macronutrient and provide energy for the body. Instead of avoiding carbohydrates altogether, focus on choosing nutrient-dense, fiber-rich sources such as fruits, vegetables, whole grains, and legumes.

**Q: What role does hydration play in weight loss?**
A: Staying hydrated is important for overall health and can support weight loss by promoting satiety, enhancing metabolism, and reducing cravings. Aim to drink plenty of water throughout the day and hydrate primarily with calorie-free beverages.

**Q: How do I deal with social events or eating out while attempting to lose weight?**
A: Plan ahead for social situations by making healthy choices, practicing portion control, and finding alternative ways to enjoy the company of others without relying on food. When dining out,

look for menu options that align with your goals and consider sharing meals or asking for modifications.

**Q: Is it necessary to track calories or macros for weight loss?**
A: While tracking calories or macros can be a useful tool for some individuals, it's not necessary for everyone. Focus on listening to your body's hunger and fullness cues, making balanced food choices, and prioritizing nutrient-dense foods.

Q: **Can stress affect weight loss efforts?**
A: Yes, chronic stress can affect weight loss efforts by increasing cortisol levels, promoting cravings for high-calorie foods, and disrupting sleep patterns. Finding healthy ways to manage stress, such as exercise, meditation, or spending time outdoors, can support weight loss goals.

www.ingramcontent.com/pod-product-compliance
Lightning Source LLC
Chambersburg PA
CBHW071029250726

48653CB00005B/1773